How to Get Rid of High Blood Pressure or Hypertension Naturally

By M. Usman

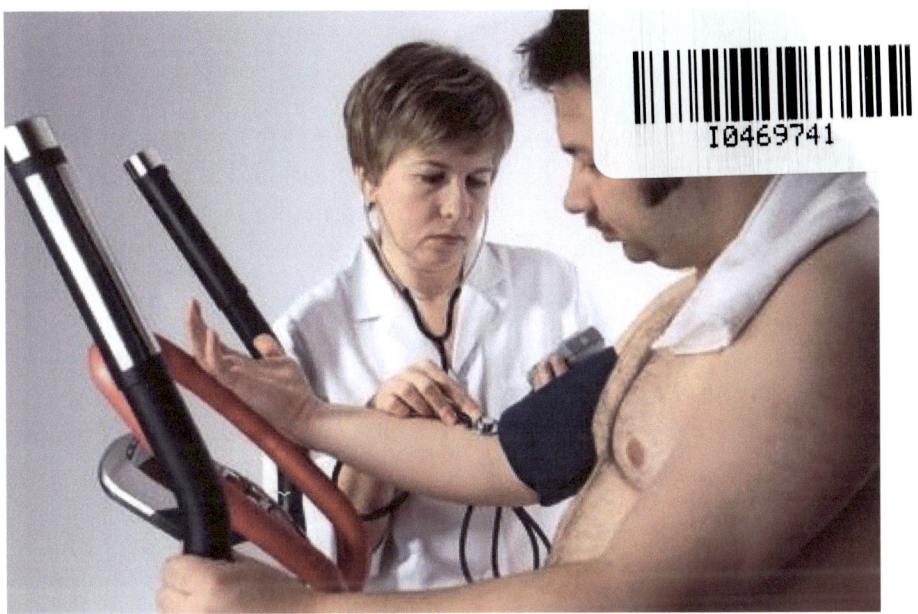

Health Learning Series

Mendon Cottage Books

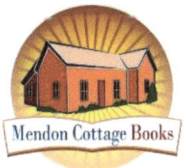

JD-Biz Publishing

Disclaimer

The information is this book is provided for informational purposes only. It is not intended to be used and medical advice or a substitute for proper medical treatment by a qualified health care provider. The information is believed to be accurate as presented based on research by the author.

The contents have not been evaluated by the U.S. Food and Drug Administration or any other Government or Health Organization and the contents in this book are not to be used to treat cure or prevent disease.

The author or publisher are not responsible for the use or safety of any diet, procedure or treatment mentioned in this book. The author or publisher is not responsible for errors or omissions that may exist.

Warning

The Book is for informational purposes only and before taking on any diet, treatment or medical procedure it is recommended to consult with your primary care provider.

Our books are available at

1. Amazon.com

2. Barnes and Noble

3. Itunes

4. Kobo

5. Smashwords

6. Google Play Books

Table of Contents

Introduction

"In the United States, about 77.9 million (1 out of 3) adults have high blood pressure." (American Heart Association, 2013 fact sheet)

According to the same report, the prevalence of hypertension in the United States population is likely to increase by 7.2% in 2030 as compared to 2013. The American population spends a total of 52 billion $ for the treatment of hypertension and its associated complications. Hypertension is reported as one of the leading causes of death throughout the world. The death toll has significantly increased due to the hypertension induced stroke and heart attack.

"In the United States, about 69% of people who have a first heart attack, 77% who have a first stroke, and 74% who have a first congestive heart failure have blood pressure higher than 140/90 mmHg." (American Heart Association, 2013 fact sheet)

So, cure of hypertension is essential for healthy living and increasing life expectancy. If you are looking for effective remedies for hypertension, then "How to get rid of hypertension? Read Now!" is the book you need. This book gives a detailed yet quick review of all the homemade, herbal, allopathic and surgical remedies for hypertension.

Each chapter of this book gives you a deep insight to the basic causes of hypertension and helps answer your basic question: "How to get rid of hypertension?"

Following the guidelines regarding the life style changes, eating habits, herbal and homemade remedies, and allopathic treatments, mentioned in this book, you can overcome this problem in a quick and effective manner and can prevent the relapse of symptoms.

Section one- Knowing hypertension.

What is hypertension?

Blood pressure, also known as mean arterial pressure, is one of the vital signs of human body. Each part of the human body requires a continuous supply of nutrients and oxygen. These components are supplied by the circulating blood. Heart is the basic organ responsible for the pumping of blood. When heart pumps blood into the blood vessels, the circulating blood exerts some pressure on the walls of vessels. This force exerted is known as blood pressure. In other words, blood pressure is the pressure exerted by circulation blood on the walls of blood vessels. During each heart beat, the blood pressure changes from maximum value (systolic pressure) to the minimum value (diastolic pressure). This difference in the pressure is responsible for the flow of blood through the tissues of human body.

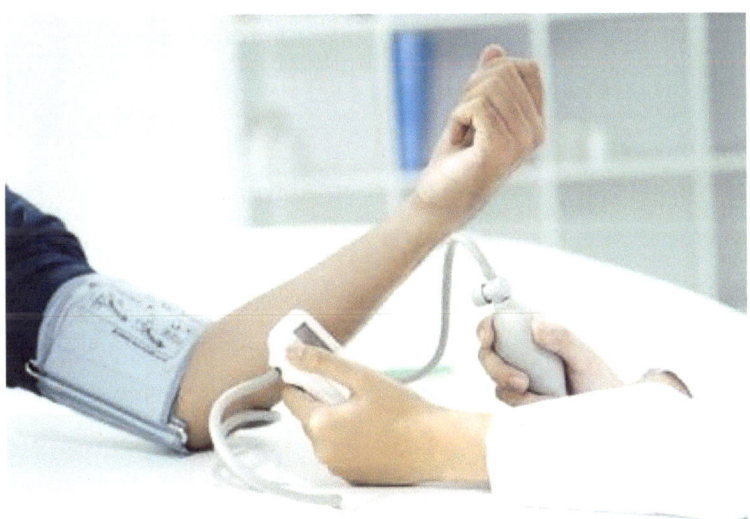

You can't just feel your blood pressure like other vital signs i.e. respiratory rate, temperature etc. You've to measure your blood pressure with the help of manual or electronic sphygmomanometer. This instrument measures the blood pressure in "millimeter of mercury mmHg". The normal of blood pressure is 120/80 mmHg. Where, 120 mmHg is the systolic or higher blood pressure and 80mmHg is the diastolic or lower blood pressure.

Now, a question comes to mind: "what is hypertension or high blood pressure?" Hypertension doesn't presents with some obvious symptoms unlike the fluctuations in other vital signs of body. For example an increase in the temperature in the body presents itself in the form of obvious symptoms like fever and lethargy. Then what is the way to know if you have hypertension or not? The only way to know this is to measure your blood pressure on regular basis. A simple table can help you access your blood pressure status:

➢ 80/120 mmHg --- Normal blood pressure.
➢ 80-90/120-135 mmHg --- Pre-hypertension.
➢ >90/140 mmHg ---- Hypertension.
➢ 90-100/140-160 mmHg --- Stage 1 hypertension.
➢ >100/160 mmHg ----- Stage 2 hypertension.

Hypertension is either of primary/ essential type or of secondary type. Primary hypertension accounts for more than 90% of all the hypertension and is due to idiopathic, unknown, causes. Secondary hypertension, accounting for about 10% of hypertension, is due to the improper function of kidney, heart, arteries and endocrine system.

Do you have hypertension? - Access by Symptoms.

- **Symptoms in primary hypertension:**

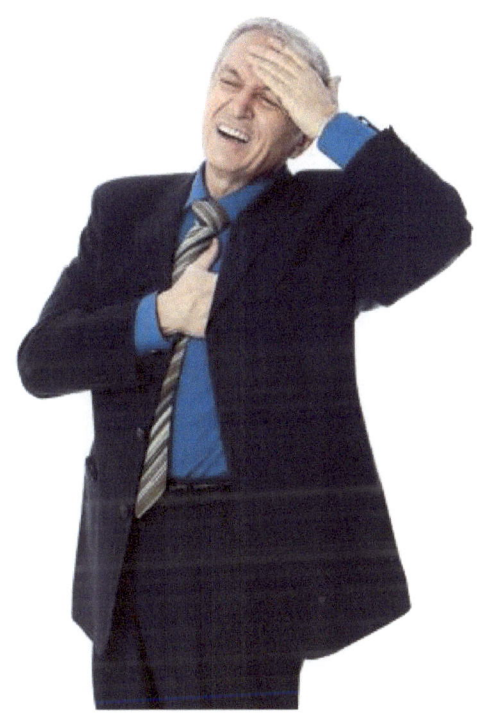

Primary or idiopathic hypertension rarely shows some obvious symptoms. The only way to access hypertension in such conditions is to monitor the blood pressure closely. However, primary hypertension may present itself in the form of multiple signs like:

- ✓ Headache.
- ✓ Light headedness.
- ✓ Buzzing sound in the ear.

✓ Loss of balance.

✓ Poor vision.

✓ Fainting.

✓ Anxiety.

✓ Body aches and fatigue.

Symptoms in secondary hypertension:

However, secondary hypertension shows multiple signs and is easy to diagnose. The major symptoms in such cases include:

✓ Cushing's syndrome i.e. an abnormality of adrenal gland causing an abnormal release of steroids into the blood leading to the increase in blood pressure, shows characteristic symptoms like obesity, glucose intolerance, moon like shape and buffalo like torso.

✓ Goiter is also followed by hypertension and shows several distinct signs like muscle tremors, anxiety, diarrhea, increased body temperature, increased appetite and muscle wasting.

✓ An increase in the release of growth hormones i.e. acromegaly, is also associated with hypertension. The symptoms in this case include enlarged face and tongue, webbed hands and feet and increased size of the visceras.

✓ Renal artery stenosis i.e. narrowing of renal artery, is an important cause of hypertension. Any abnormal sound in the blood vessels increases the suspicion of this abnormality.

✓ Coarctation of aorta i.e. narrowing of aorta, can cause severe hypertension in the upper extremities of human body. A delay or complete absence of femoral artery pulsation strongly advocates the presence of this condition.

✓ Pheochromocytoma i.e. an abnormally high titer of catecholamines, can cause severe hypertension. Any symptom like headache, pallor, palpitations etc. strongly suggests the presence of this abnormality.

Symptoms in hypertensive crisis:

Hypertensive crisis is a medical emergency when the blood pressure shoots to an abnormal value of 180/110 mmHg. It's a dangerous condition as prolong exposure to this condition can cause drastic outcomes like blindness, stroke and heart failure. So, this condition needs immediate rectification. There is a specific pattern of symptoms related to hypertensive crisis:

✓ Headache.
✓ Extreme blurring of vision.
✓ Absolute loss of consciousness.
✓ Difficulty in breathing.

Symptoms in pregnancy:

Hypertension is a common side effect of **pregnancy**. Almost 8-10% of the pregnant women experience hypertension of varying degree. The symptoms of hypertension in pregnant women include:

✓ Visual disturbance.
✓ Edema.

✓ Vomiting.

✓ Pain in the abdomen.

✓ Death of the infant.

✓ Death of the mother in extreme cases.

Symptoms in children:

In **children**, the symptoms of hypertension vary as:

✓ Failure of normal growth.

✓ Irritability.

✓ Lack of physical and mental strength.

✓ Seizures.

✓ Difficulty in breathing.

✓ Headache.

✓ Bleeding of nose or gums.

✓ Poor vision.

✓ Fatigue.

What causes hypertension?

There are two basic types of hypertension:

➤ Essential or primary hypertension.
➤ Secondary hypertension.

Essential or primary hypertension:
Essential or primary hypertension causes almost 90% of all the hypertensive conditions. In essential hypertension, there is an increase in the blood pressure without an obvious medical cause. However, several factors contribute the development of primary hypertension:

✓ Aging is one of the most important causes that contribute to the development of essential hypertension. Aging compromises the function of heart and makes the vessels hard and non-compliant. These factors, in turn ,cause hypertension.
✓ Life style is another important determinant of essential hypertension. People that don't involve themselves in physical activities are more prone to the development of hypertension.
✓ Eating habits, sometimes, also contribute to the development of high blood pressure. High salt intake, high cholesterol intake, eating food low in dietary fibers, low intake of vitamin E etc. can contribute to the development of hypertension.
✓ Generic factors also play an important role. The hereditary predisposition to hypertension is still a poorly understood phenomenon. However, several studies confirm that cardiovascular problems mostly run in families.

- ✓ Stress is extremely important in developing high blood pressure. It has been observed that people that remain stressed all the times are more prone to the detrimental effects high blood pressure.
- ✓ Several environmental factors also contribute the development of hypertension.

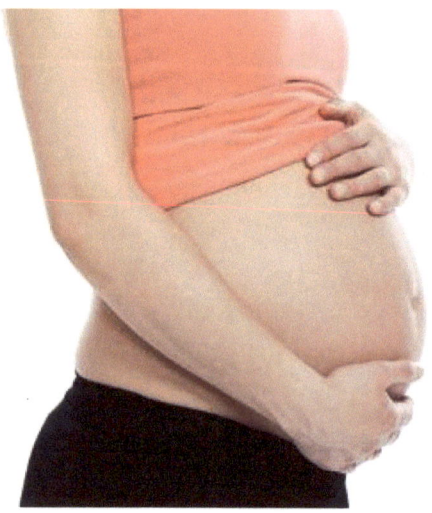

Secondary hypertension:

Secondary hypertension constitutes almost 5-10% of all the hypertensions. Secondary hypertension develops due to identifiable reasons. The basic causes of secondary hypertension include:

- ✓ Pregnancy is one of the most important physiological causes of hypertension. High blood pressure develops in pregnancy due to hormonal disturbance.
- ✓ Hyper or hypo thyroidism also increase the chances of hypertension.

- ✓ Coarctation of aorta may cause high blood pressure.
- ✓ Pheochromocytoma is an important cause of hypertension.

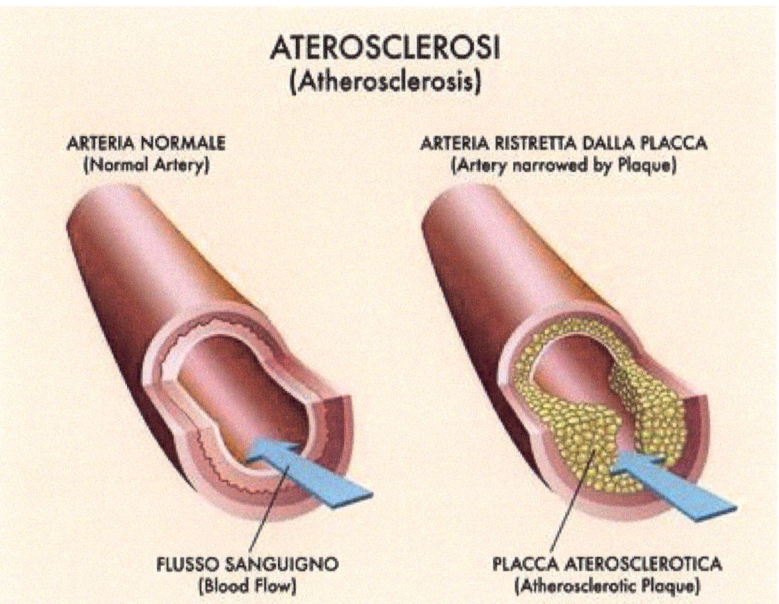

- ✓ Hyperaldestronism i.e. an increase in the release of aldosterone, causes retention of salts and water and causes hypertension as a result.
- ✓ Cushing syndrome causes hypertension because of excessive salt and water retention.
- ✓ Atherosclerosis in the walls of blood vessels is the leading cause of deaths due to high blood pressure. Atherosclerosis causes increased deposit along the walls of blood vessels leading to the decrease in the caliber of vessels. This, in turn, causes hypertension.
- ✓ Excessive liquorice consumption may also cause hypertension.

✓ Hypertension may develop as a side effect to the use of some medicines.

Health risks due to hypertension

Uncontrolled hypertension inflicts serious stress on the walls of blood vessels and heart. Severe hypertension can lead to several health complications like:

Heart failure:

High blood pressure can cause thickening of the walls of heart, which can ultimately lead to heart failure.

Stroke:

The vessels of brain can withstand pressure only to a specific limit. When the pressure of blood in the cerebral blood vessels increases, it can cause the rupture of these vessels. This condition is known as brain hemorrhage or stroke. Brain is the center of all body activities and it requires continuous supply of blood. The supply of blood to the brain decreases as the blood vessels rupture. It can cause serious learning disabilities and physical abnormalities.

Blindness

High blood pressure can cause the rupture of blood vessels in eyes that can ultimately lead to permanent blindness.

Aneurysm of blood vessels:

When a constant stress is applied against the wall of blood vessels, they become dilated and bulging. This bulging of blood vessels is called the aneurysm of blood vessels. These vessels can rupture leading to a life threatening hemorrhage.

Kidney failure:

High blood pressure can cause the rupture of blood vessels in the kidneys leading to permanent kidney failure.

Metabolic disorders:

High blood pressure causes a cluster of metabolic disorders like:

- ✓ High triglycerides.
- ✓ Decrease HDL (good fats).
- ✓ Increased level of cholesterol.
- ✓ Increased resistance to insulin leading to an increased risk of diabetes.
- ✓ Increased risks of obesity.

Section Two- Treatments of hypertension.

Treatments of hypertension- An overview

"High blood pressure was listed as the primary cause of death in 348,102 Americans in the year 2009." *(American Heart Association)*

This makes high blood pressure an extremely dangerous condition. An uncontrolled and untreated hypertension always ends up in fatal consequences. In the last few decades, drastic changes in our life style and eating habits have increased the prevalence of high blood pressure. Eating junk food, lack of exercise, lack of social activities, too much stress and tension has increased the chances of development of high blood pressure in the common population.

High blood pressure is a silent killer because it doesn't produce any obvious symptoms unlike other medical conditions. Most of the people end up in serious medical complications because they never know that they are suffering from hypertension. This feature of hypertension, particularly, makes it extremely life threatening.

Luckily, a lot of remedies are available for the treatment of hypertension. The remedies for hypertension include:

- ✓ Several homemade remedies are available that come straight from your fridge or cupboard.
- ✓ Several herbal remedies help minimize the harmful effects of hypertension in a natural way.

- ✓ Several life style changes like regular exercise etc. can help a lot in the treatment of hypertension.
- ✓ The food you eat greatly alters your blood pressure. So, be vigilant of what you eat. Eating a healthy, cholesterol free diet, abstinence from alcohol and smoking etc. can help a lot in controlling hypertension.
- ✓ Controlling anxiety and depression can help manage hypertension as well.
- ✓ There are a large number of medicines available for the treatment of hypertension.
- ✓ Some surgical methods are also available for some kinds of hypertension.

Treat hypertension from common home stuff - home remedies

Several homemade remedies are available for hypertension that treats hypertension in an effective manner. All these remedies are natural and are without any side effect. All home remedies are cost effective and are easily available. Such homemade remedies for hypertension include:

Garlic:

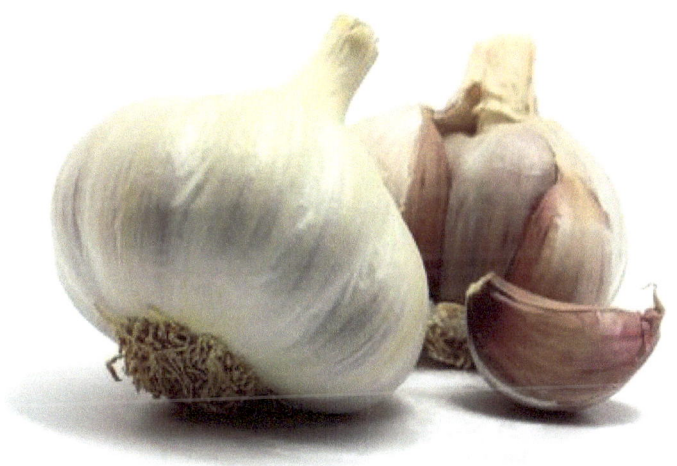

Both raw and cooked garlic are equally effective in the treatment of hypertension. Garlic is believed to reduce hypertension because of its ability to produce hydrogen sulfide. This compound not only improves the flow of blood in the body but also decreases the production of gas in stomach and thus decreases the pressure on the heart. In the case of severe hypertension, you should use 1 or 2 cloves each day. You can also add it into your diet and can also use garlic oil for better results.

Banana:

Banana is an effective homemade remedy for hypertension that you can use regularly. Banana is a rich source of potassium. Potassium helps optimize the function of heart and thus helps in the regulation of blood pressure. An additional character which makes banana an ideal food for hypertensive patients is that it contains very low level of sodium and cholesterol. Thus, it prevents the increase of blood pressure.

Lemon:

Lemon in the form of lemonades, lemon juices or other lemon drinks is advised to the patients of hypertension. It's a rich source of vitamin C that's a powerful anti-oxidant which helps improve the health of blood vessels. Moreover, it contains a high content of vitamin B which is extremely beneficial for the proper functioning of heart.

Celery:

It's a rich source of 3-butylphthalide, a type of chemical, which helps maintain the normal flow of blood through the blood vessels. Moreover, it helps reduce the level of stress hormones. A high titer of stress hormones cause constriction, which, in return, leads to an increase in the level of blood pressure.

Honey:

The beneficial effects of honey are known to all. Honey helps normalize the function of heart and also helps in optimization of the function of blood vessels. The patients of hypertension should make a habit of consuming honey on daily basis. You can eat honey as such or can add it in your morning cereals, juices and shakes. You can also make a tea by adding garlic and a tea spoon of honey. The sugars in honey are easily metabolized and also don't alter the sugar level in the blood.

Onion juice:

Onion juice is another effective homemade remedy for hypertension. You can eat a raw medium sized onion or you can add it into your meals. You can also make a paste by mixing half tea spoon of both honey and onion juice. Consume this juice twice each day.

Coconut water:

Dirking coconut water provides you with several vial nutrients like potassium. Potassium helps improve the function of both heart and blood vessels. So, drinking coconut water, in addition to water, is a good idea for hypertensive patients.

Cayenne pepper:

People suffering from mild degrees of hypertension should consume cayenne pepper on daily basis. This ingredient helps prevent the accumulation of platelets in the blood vessels and can thus help in the smooth circulation of blood in the body. Add this pepper into your daily meals, salads and soups for optimum results.

Watermelon seeds:

All parts of watermelon are unique in their beneficial features. The seeds of watermelon, in particular, are very useful for the patients of hypertension. So, make these seeds a part of your diet plan.

Fenugreek seeds:

Take a spoon full of these seeds and boil them in water for 2 minutes. Remove the seeds from the water and blend these seeds in a blender. Use this paste twice a day for better results.

Try some herbs

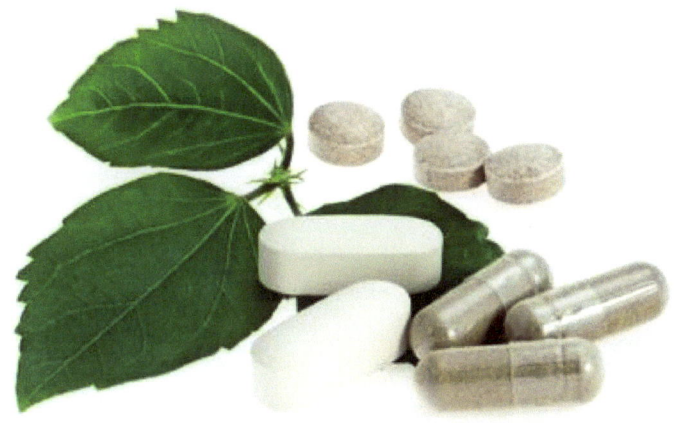

The focus of therapy is now shifting from allopathic medicines to the herbal medicines because herbal medicines provide an effective cure of medical condition and are without serious side effects. All these remedies are based on the use of leaf, shoots, roots, flowers, seeds and fruits of plants, trees and bushes. Nature has provided a wide variety of herbs that are seen to reduce elevated blood pressure and also help decrease the chances of cardiovascular events. Moreover, these herbs are cost effective and are easily available. All the allopathic medicines have well documented side effects. But, natural herbs are without serious side effects are much safe to use. Different herbs used in the treatment of hypertension include:

Prickly custard apple:

It's a natural herb that belongs to the family of custard apple trees. The scientific name of this herb is Annona muricata. The leaf extracts of this plant help reduce high blood pressure and help improve the function of both heart and blood vessels.

Breadfruit:
This herb is very effective in neutralizing the effect of catecholamine i.e. natural substances that increase blood pressure by constricting blood vessels and increasing the heart rate. The use of this herb helps neutralize increase in the blood pressure induced by catecholamine in experimental animals.

Green oats:
It helps normalize the levels of both sugar and cholesterol, an increase level of which can cause increase in blood pressure. Moreover, it helps improve the efficiency of heart function.

Green tea:
Green tea is very beneficial for the treatment of hypertension. It's rich in anti-oxidants and thus helps prevent the damage to the heart and blood vessels induced by oxygen free radicals. It also improves the heart function and decreases the chances of heart attack.

Hawthorn:
This is a Chinese herb that's reported to decrease blood pressure. This blood pressure reducing effect of hawthorn is because of two of its ingredients: flavonoids and procyanidins, which are both excellent anti-oxidants. This herb decreases the probability of clot formation and decreases the chances of heart attack.

Lavender oil:

This oil is mainly used for massaging the body and head. This oil has great relaxant properties and helps reduce stress- one of the basic reasons of hypertension.

Basil:

Basil leaves have got anti-hypertensive effects. This effect of basil is attributed to the presence of certain chemicals that help block calcium channels in the walls of blood vessels leading to the relaxation of blood vessels and decrease in blood pressure.

Sesame:

The extracts obtained from sesame seeds are proved to reduce blood pressure. This anti-hypertensive effect of sesame seeds is due to the presence of acetylcholine like substances that help cause the relaxation of blood vessels in reduction in heart rate.

Coca beans:

These beans are used for the production of coffee, cocoa powder and chocolates. The active ingredient of these beans is flavonoids. Flavonoids stimulate the release of nitric oxide, which causes an increase in the caliber of blood vessels. This causes a significant decrease in hypertension.

Ginger:

Ginger is an extremely beneficial herb that has been long used because of its beneficial effects. It has got powerful anti-oxidant properties, helps in metabolizing fat and sugar and decreases the chances of cardio-vascular events. You can add it into your tea or can add it into your daily meals.

Change your life style

In most of the cases, the basic cause of hypertension is as simple as an improper lifestyle. Decreased physical activities, eating junk food, smoking, alcohol intake and excessive stress cause an increase in the blood pressure. In such conditions, simple life style changes can help a lot in curing hypertension. Such life style changes include:

Lose extra weight:

Fat deposits in the walls of blood vessels cause an increase in the blood pressure. So, losing extra fat can help a lot in getting rid of hypertension. Losing just 10 pounds of your weight can help normalize your blood pressure. In other words, more weight you lose, the better effects you get. The beneficial effects of medicines are also optimized by reducing blood pressure.

Besides, too much fat around your waistline can increase the chances of development of hypertension. So, keep a close eye on your waistline. In general:

- ✓ Men with a waist of 40 inch or above are prone to the development of hypertension and cardiovascular event.
- ✓ Women with a waist of 35or above are at a high risk.

Regular exercise:

Simple exercises like aerobics, swimming, cycling, jogging or brisk walking are very beneficial for the patients of hypertension. If you are a patient of pre-hypertension then regular exercise can help prevent the development of hypertension. On the other hand, if you are a patient of hypertension then regular exercise can help reduce your blood pressure to safer limits.

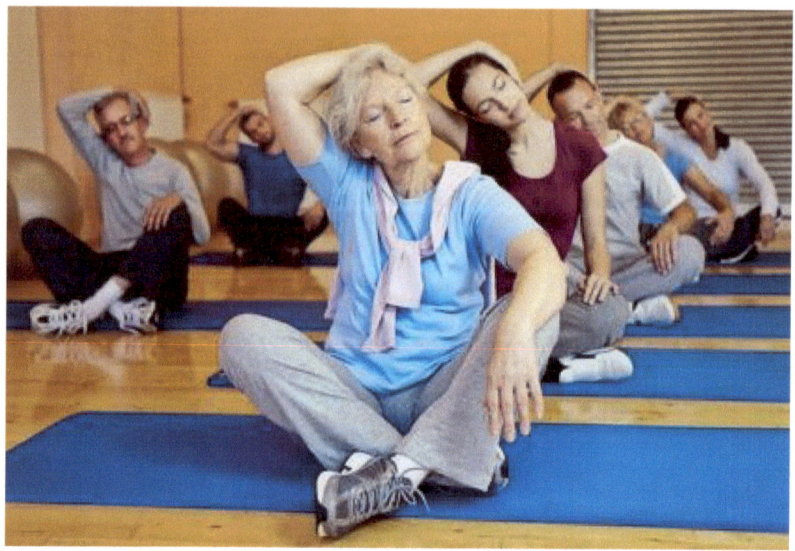

Exercise helps reduce blood pressure because of its following effects:

- ✓ It reduces stress.
- ✓ It helps burn fats and cholesterol.
- ✓ It keeps the blood sugar level within a normal range.
- ✓ It helps improve the flow of blood to all parts of body.

Healthy diet:

Life these days has become very fast and people haven't got enough time to put together a healthy diet plan. People prefer food which they can eat on the go. That's why the use of junk food has become very popular. But, the use of fast food has demented our health and one serious health complication we face is hypertension. So, simple improvement in eating habits can help in curing hypertension. Such changes include:

✓ Keep a record of what you eat. At the end of the week, access the eating habits that are harmful and try to minimize those habits.
✓ Try improving the intake of potassium.
✓ Always read the labels of food products you buy. Design a healthy and balanced diet plan.

Reduce sodium intake.

Increased sodium intake is one of the most important causes of hypertension. When the intake of sodium is very high, the kidneys conserve this sodium and water along with this sodium. This results in an increase in the volume of blood and increase in the blood pressure. So, reducing your sodium intake to as much 2300 mg per day can help reduce 2-10 mmHg of blood pressure. You can minimize the sodium intake by:

✓ Reading the labels of food products before you buy them.
✓ Minimizing the use of sodium in your diet, drinks and salads.
✓ Eating fewer processed foods as they have a high content of sodium in them.

Reduce alcohol intake:

Chronic intake of alcohol can cause health complications like liver damage, high blood pressure and increased risk of stroke and heart attack. So, giving up the habit of alcohol intake can help reduce as much as 10 mmHg of your blood pressure.

Avoid smoking:

An intact endothelium (lining) of blood vessels is required in order to maintain a normal caliber of blood vessels. However, chronic smoking can damage this endothelium and causes high blood pressure and increased risks of heart attack. So, try to quit smoking. Medicines like veranicline, nicotine chew gums and nicotine patches can also be used for this purpose.

Be careful of what you eat

Eating habits are one of the basic determinants in the treatment of hypertension. A healthy, balanced and well planned diet plan can greatly lower the blood pressure and can reduce the chances of stroke and heart attack. The diet plan for hypertension should contain following important components:

Whole grains:
A balanced, anti-hypertensive diet should contain whole grains like oat meal. These grains are rich in fibers, magnesium and potassium. All these nutrients are very beneficial in the treatment of high blood pressure.

Olive oil:
Animal fats are high in saturated (bad fats). Use of these oils for cooking purposes can increase the levels of cholesterol inside the body.

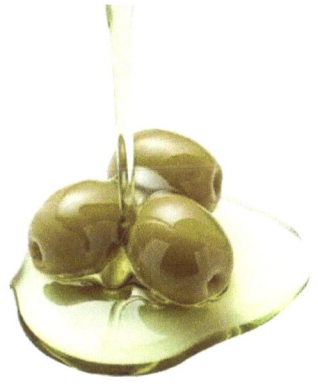

This high level of cholesterol, in turn, leads to an increase deposit along the walls of blood vessels causing hypertension. So, plant oils should be used instead of animal oils for cooking purposes. Olive oil is one of the best plant oils that hypertensive patients can use. Not only is it low in fats but is also rich in anti-oxidants. So, it helps a great deal in minimizing the blood pressure.

Ground flaxseeds:

Add flaxseed in your diet. These seeds are rich in omega-3 fatty acids (good fats). These fats have excellent anti-oxidant properties and are also very beneficial in conditions of inflammation and infection.

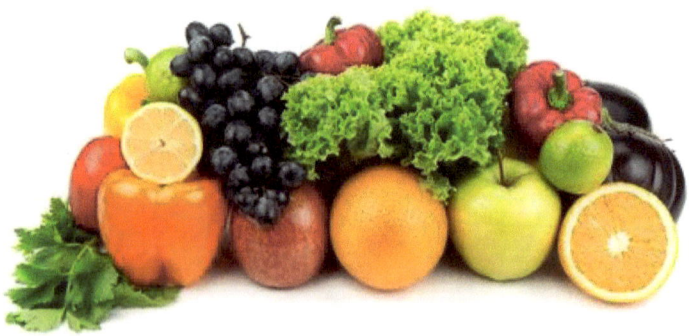

Bananas:

Bananas are one of the most important fruits that should be used by hypertensive patients on regular basis. Bananas are rich in potassium, which helps improve the function of heart and blood vessels.

Potatoes:

Potatoes have several properties that make them perfect for the patients of hypertension. Like :

✓ They are rich in magnesium, which is beneficial.

✓ They are a rich source of potassium.

✓ They are very low in sodium.

✓ They are rich in carbohydrates but poor in cholesterols.

Apricots:

Apricots, especially dry, are exceedingly beneficial for the use of hypertensive people. They are also rich in fiber, which assists in normal digestion.

Pumpkin seeds:

Make pumpkin seeds an essential component of your daily diet. These seeds are a rich source of zinc. Zinc helps improve the health of walls of blood vessels and is required for the normal function of heart.

Garlic:

Garlic is long known because of its beneficial effects on health. It has got a strong anti-oxidant property and is anti-septic in nature. Consume 1,2 cloves of garlic each day or add garlic in your daily meals or salads.

Broccoli:

Broccoli is a rich source of proteins, fibers, vitamin C and A, chromium and is low in cholesterol. These properties make it an excellent diet for the people suffering from hypertension.

Medicines for hypertension- An effective remedy.

Though homemade remedies, herbal treatment, life style changes and dietary restriction can help in controlling hypertension but they can't cure the underlying cause of hypertension. So, the use of medicines is inevitable, or one should say necessary, for a permanent cure of hypertension. Several medicines are available that have proved to be extremely beneficial in the treatment of hypertension. However, all these medicines should be used after the recommendation of physician, Self medication should be avoided as it does more harm than good. Diuretic drugs include:

Diuretics:

Diuretic, also known as water pills, decrease blood pressure by causing elimination of extra salts and water. This loss of water and salts, in turn, causes a decrease in blood volume, which causes a decrease in blood pressure. Such drugs include:

- ✓ Thaizide diuretic.
- ✓ Loop diuretic.
- ✓ Potassium sparing diuretics.
- ✓ Carbonic anhydrase inhibitor.

Beta blockers:

Propranolol is the prototype of this group. These drugs block the beta receptors on heart and cause a decrease in the rate and force of heart contraction.

Calcium channel blockers:

This group includes drugs like nifedipine and diltiazim. These drugs block the calcium ion channels in the walls of blood vessels and heart, causing relaxation of blood vessels and decrease in heart rate respectively. This, in turn, causes a decrease in blood presser.

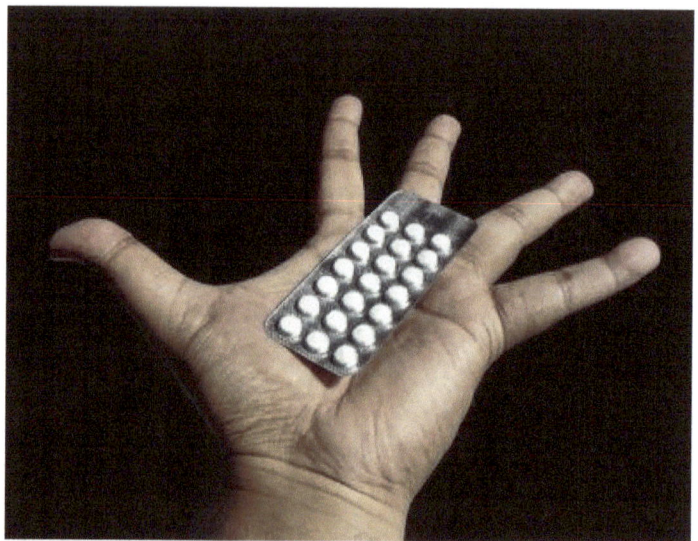

ACE inhibitors:

Angiotensin is a hormone released by kidneys which is responsible for the contraction of blood vessels and water and salt retention by kidneys. Angiotensin converting enzyme inhibitor drugs, like captopril, inhibit the synthesis of angiotensin and thus help decreased blood pressure.

Angiotensin receptor blockers:

The effect of angiotensin of its receptors is blocked by this group of drugs. This group includes dugs like losartan.

Aldosterone receptor blockers:

Aldosterone is a steroid hormone which acts on kidney and causes it to conserve water and salts. However, this effect of aldosterone is blocked by aldosterone receptor blockers. This group includes drugs like spironolactone and eplerenone.

Vasodilators:

This group includes drugs like minoxidil sulfate. These drugs cause a decrease in the tone of vascular smooth muscles leading to a significant decrease in blood vessels.

Alpha blockers:

Clomifine and methyl dopa is a member of this group. These drugs block the alpha receptors present on the walls of blood vessels leading to the relaxation of wall of blood vessels and decrease in blood pressure.

Surgical correction of hypertension

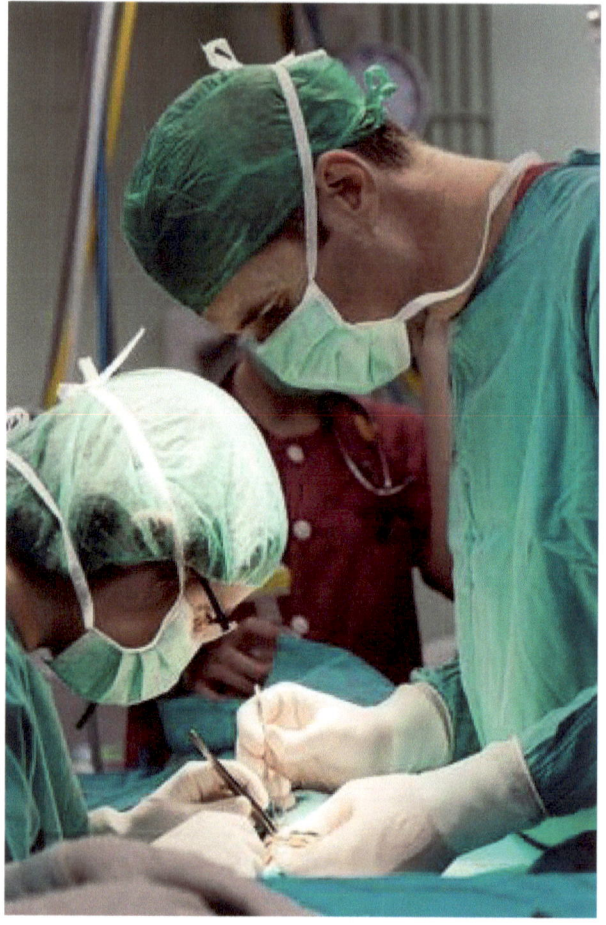

This type of treatment is beneficial only in the case of secondary hypertension, when a specific medical cause is known. Following are the conditions in which surgical correction can help cure hypertension:

✓ If hypertension is due to hyperthyroidism, then the condition can be cured by the surgical removal of thyroid.

- ✓ If the condition is secondary to the development of a tumor in pituitary gland, then surgery can used to remove this tumor.
- ✓ Similar, surgery can be used for the removal of tumors in adrenal gland.
- ✓ Any coarctation of aorta or major blood vessels can also be corrected surgically.
- ✓ Extra fat can be removed through liposuction.

Photo credits

All Images Licensed by Fotolia.com

PhysiotherapeutinhilftSeniorenbeimHanteltraining

© Robert Kneschke - Fotolia.com

Surgery operation

© Franck Boston - Fotolia.com

set of different fruits and vegetables

© alinamd - Fotolia.com

A medicinal tablet strip in a hand of a person.

© Yogesh More - Fotolia.com

Natural pills with green leaf

© Chariclo - Fotolia.com

Heart attack

© Ana BlazicPavlovic - Fotolia.com

GruppebeimRückentrainingimFitnesscenter

© Robert Kneschke - Fotolia.com

olive oil condiment vegeterian food

© picsfive - Fotolia.com

knoblauchkollen

© Schlierner - Fotolia.com

Aterosclerosi

© rob3000 - Fotolia.com

Beautiful pregnant belly

© SergejsRahunoks - Fotolia.com

Checking blood pressure

© DragonImages - Fotolia.

Author Bio

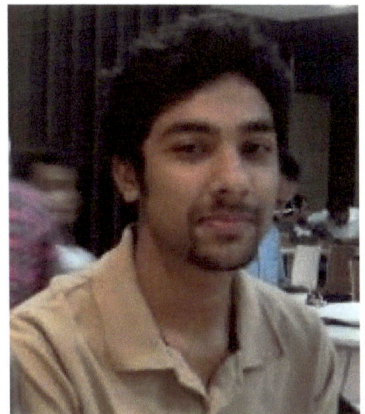

Muhammad Usman is a distinguished medical graduate of Allama iqbal medical college (AIMC). He is a professional writer who has been in the field for more than 4 years. During this time he has produced 10,000+ articles, blogs and eBooks on various niches related to diseases, health, fitness, nutrition and well being. He is a regular contributor to several journals related to medicine and surgery. He is the editor of several journals and newspapers.

Check out some of the other JD-Biz Publishing books

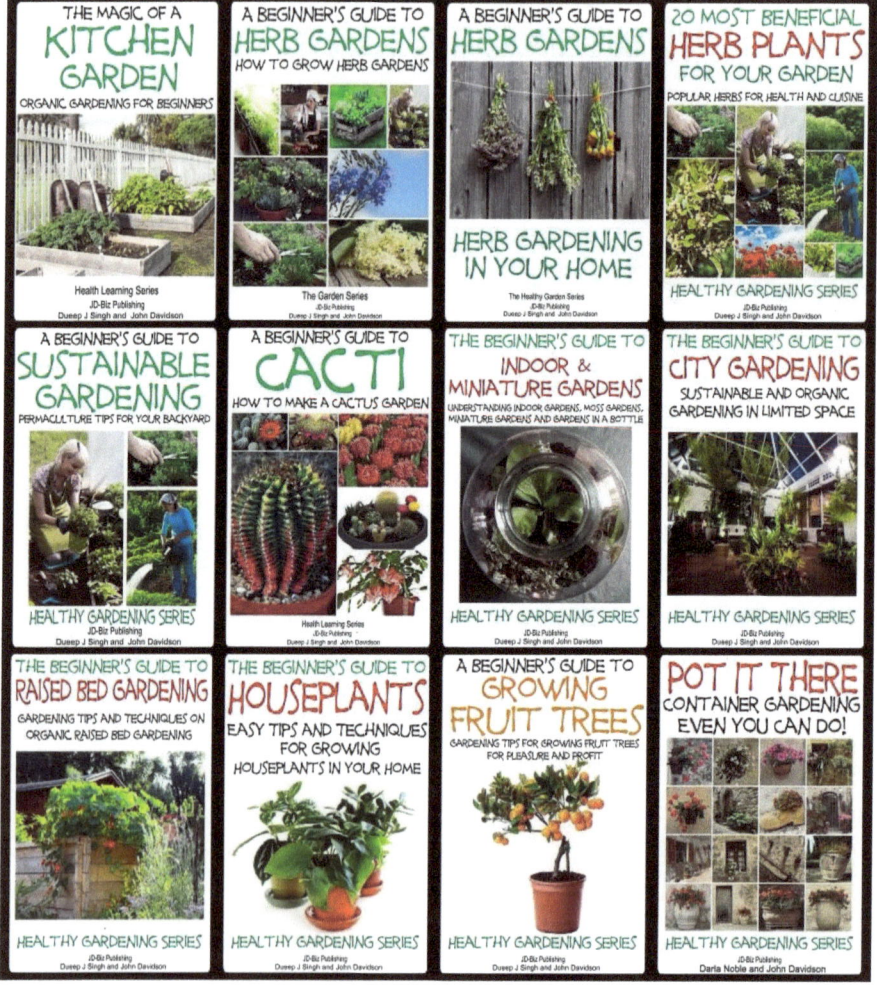

Health Learning Series

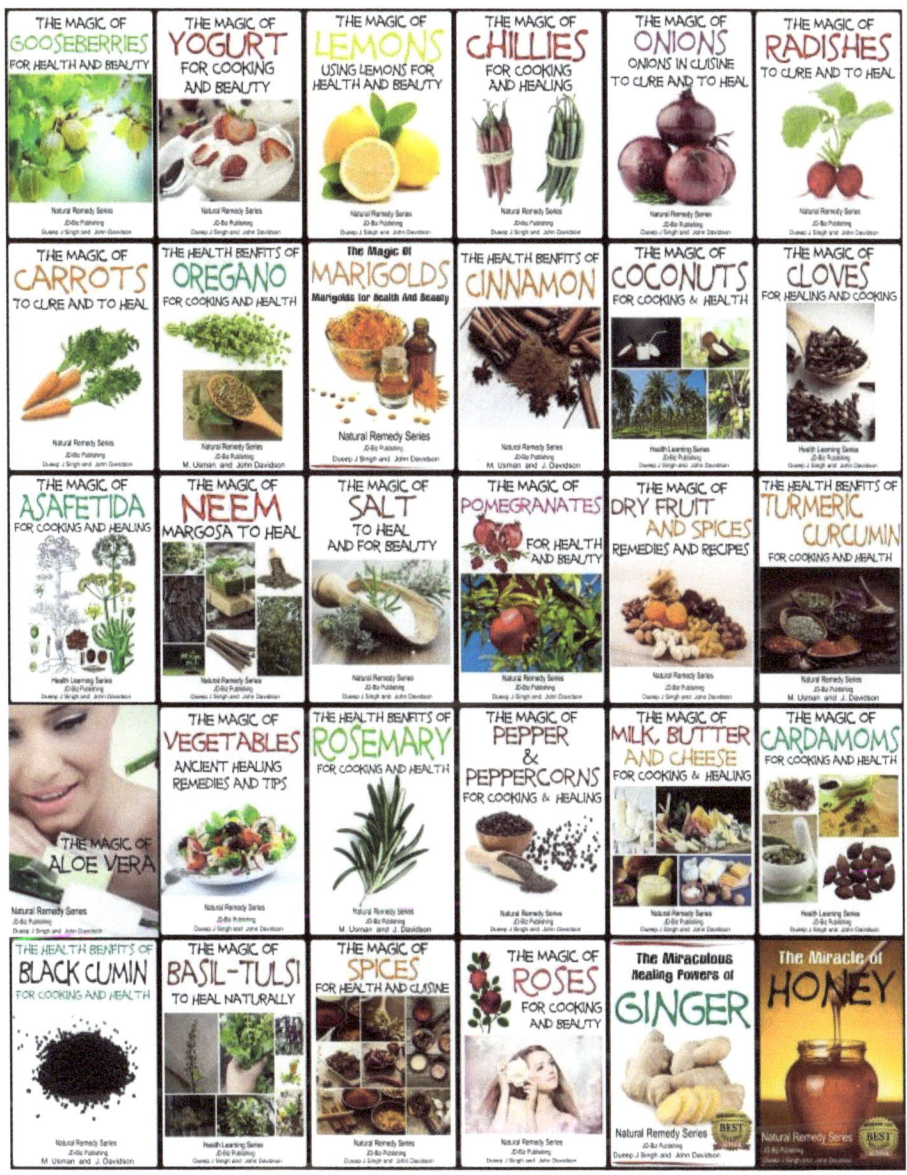

Country Life Books

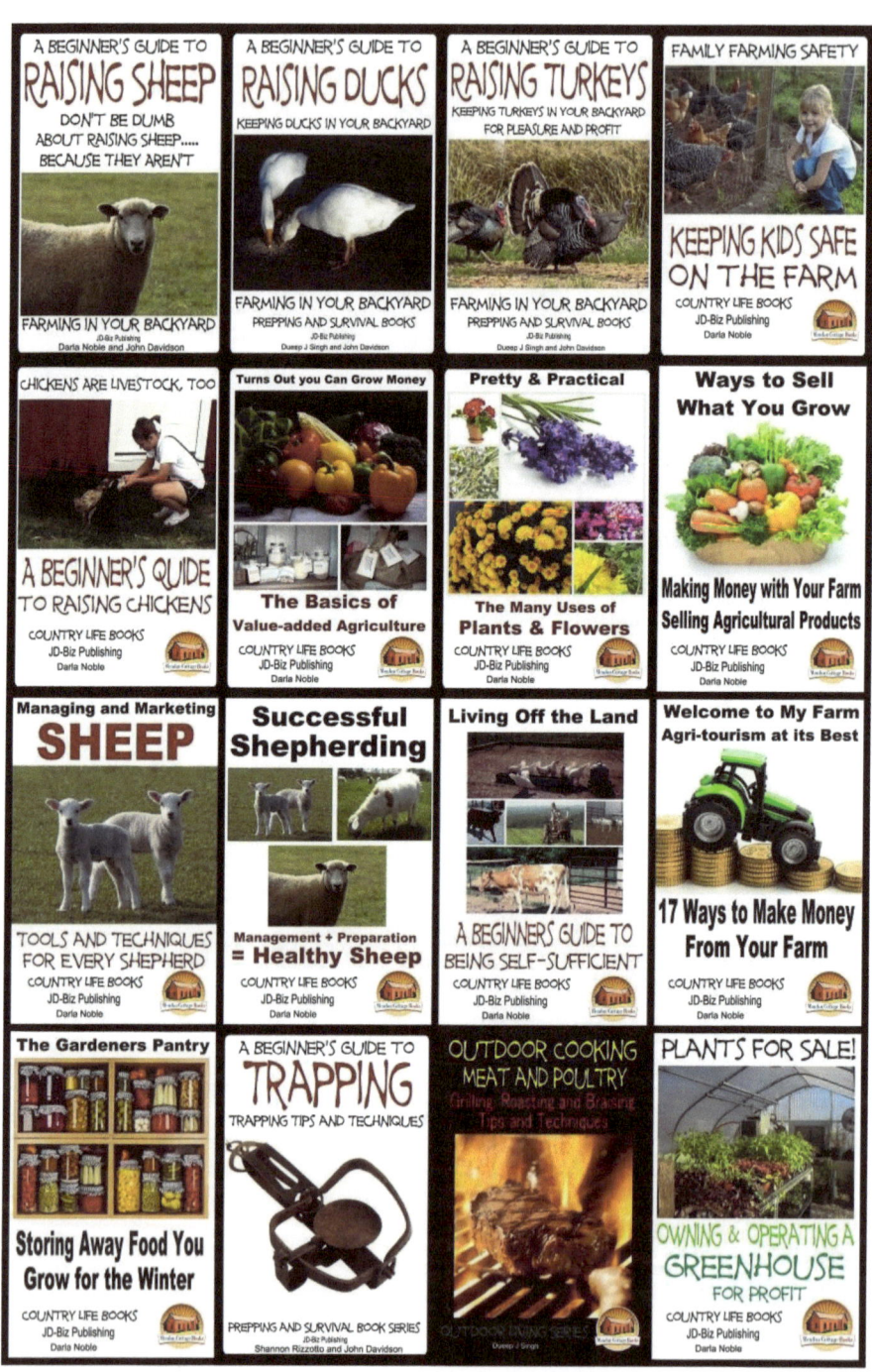

A BEGINNER'S GUIDE TO
RAISING SHEEP
DON'T BE DUMB
ABOUT RAISING SHEEP.....
BECAUSE THEY AREN'T
FARMING IN YOUR BACKYARD
JD-Biz Publishing
Darla Noble and John Davidson

A BEGINNER'S GUIDE TO
RAISING DUCKS
KEEPING DUCKS IN YOUR BACKYARD
FARMING IN YOUR BACKYARD
PREPPING AND SURVIVAL BOOKS
JD-Biz Publishing
Dueep J Singh and John Davidson

A BEGINNER'S GUIDE TO
RAISING TURKEYS
KEEPING TURKEYS IN YOUR BACKYARD
FOR PLEASURE AND PROFIT
FARMING IN YOUR BACKYARD
PREPPING AND SURVIVAL BOOKS
JD-Biz Publishing
Dueep J Singh and John Davidson

FAMILY FARMING SAFETY
**KEEPING KIDS SAFE
ON THE FARM**
COUNTRY LIFE BOOKS
JD-Biz Publishing
Darla Noble

CHICKENS ARE LIVESTOCK, TOO
**A BEGINNER'S GUIDE
TO RAISING CHICKENS**
COUNTRY LIFE BOOKS
JD-Biz Publishing
Darla Noble

Turns Out you Can Grow Money
**The Basics of
Value-added Agriculture**
COUNTRY LIFE BOOKS
JD-Biz Publishing
Darla Noble

Pretty & Practical
**The Many Uses of
Plants & Flowers**
COUNTRY LIFE BOOKS
JD-Biz Publishing
Darla Noble

**Ways to Sell
What You Grow**
**Making Money with Your Farm
Selling Agricultural Products**
COUNTRY LIFE BOOKS
JD-Biz Publishing
Darla Noble

**Managing and Marketing
SHEEP**
TOOLS AND TECHNIQUES
FOR EVERY SHEPHERD
COUNTRY LIFE BOOKS
JD-Biz Publishing
Darla Noble

**Successful
Shepherding**
Management + Preparation
= **Healthy Sheep**
COUNTRY LIFE BOOKS
JD-Biz Publishing
Darla Noble

Living Off the Land
A BEGINNERS GUIDE TO
BEING SELF-SUFFICIENT
COUNTRY LIFE BOOKS
JD-Biz Publishing
Darla Noble

**Welcome to My Farm
Agri-tourism at its Best**
**17 Ways to Make Money
From Your Farm**
COUNTRY LIFE BOOKS
JD-Biz Publishing
Darla Noble

The Gardeners Pantry
**Storing Away Food You
Grow for the Winter**
COUNTRY LIFE BOOKS
JD-Biz Publishing
Darla Noble

A BEGINNER'S GUIDE TO
TRAPPING
TRAPPING TIPS AND TECHNIQUES
PREPPING AND SURVIVAL BOOK SERIES
JD-Biz Publishing
Shannon Rizzotto and John Davidson

**OUTDOOR COOKING
MEAT AND POULTRY**
Grilling, Roasting and Braising
Tips and Techniques
OUTDOOR LIVING SERIES
Dueep J Singh

PLANTS FOR SALE!
**OWNING & OPERATING A
GREENHOUSE
FOR PROFIT**
COUNTRY LIFE BOOKS
JD-Biz Publishing
Darla Noble

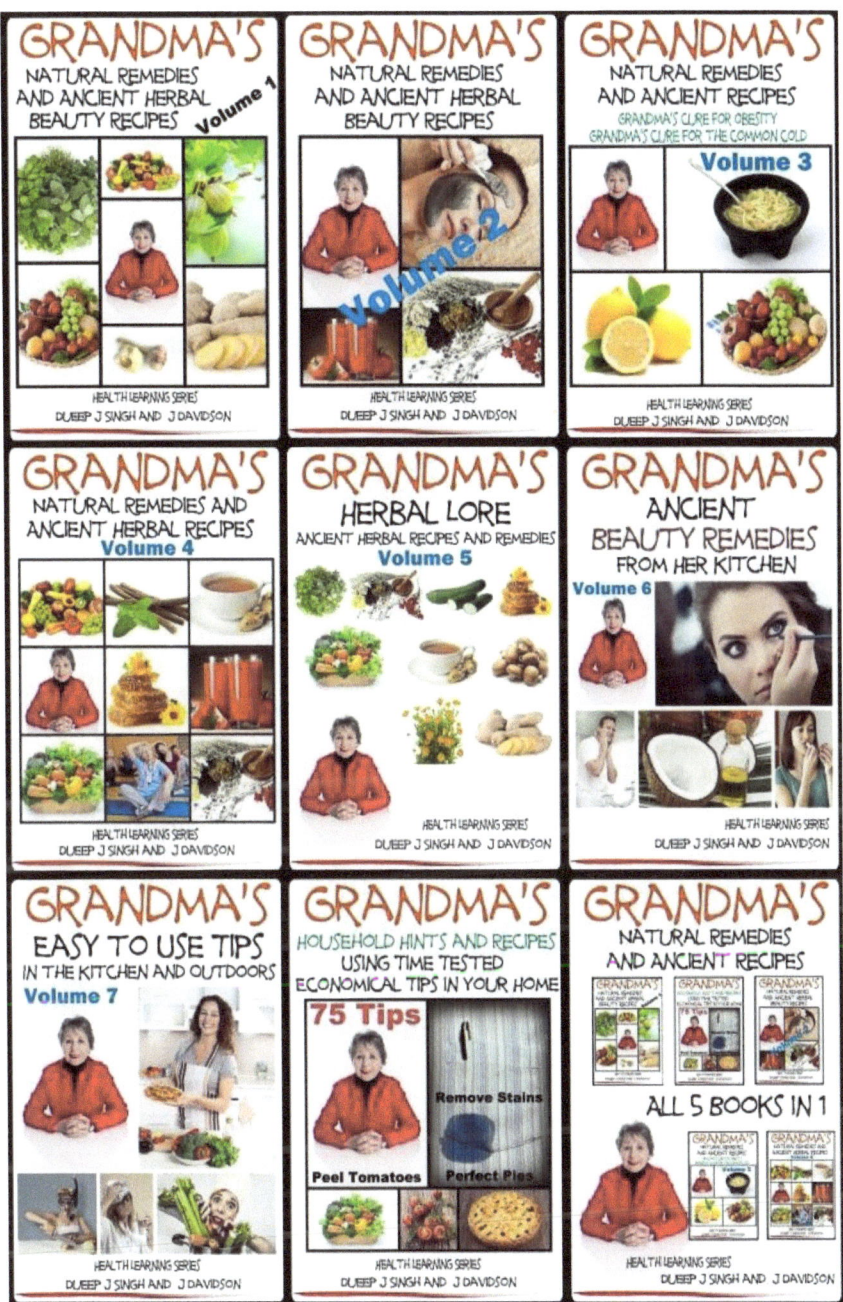

Health Learning Series

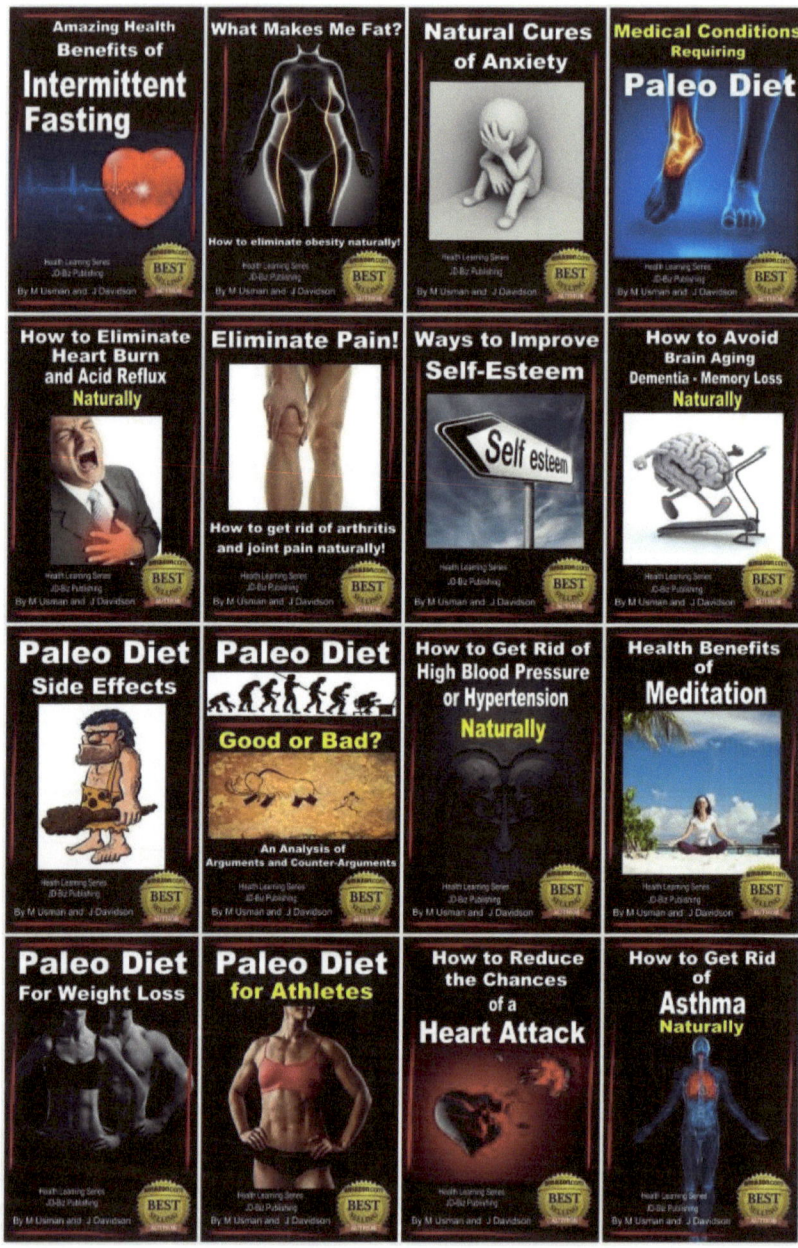

Amazing Animal Book Series

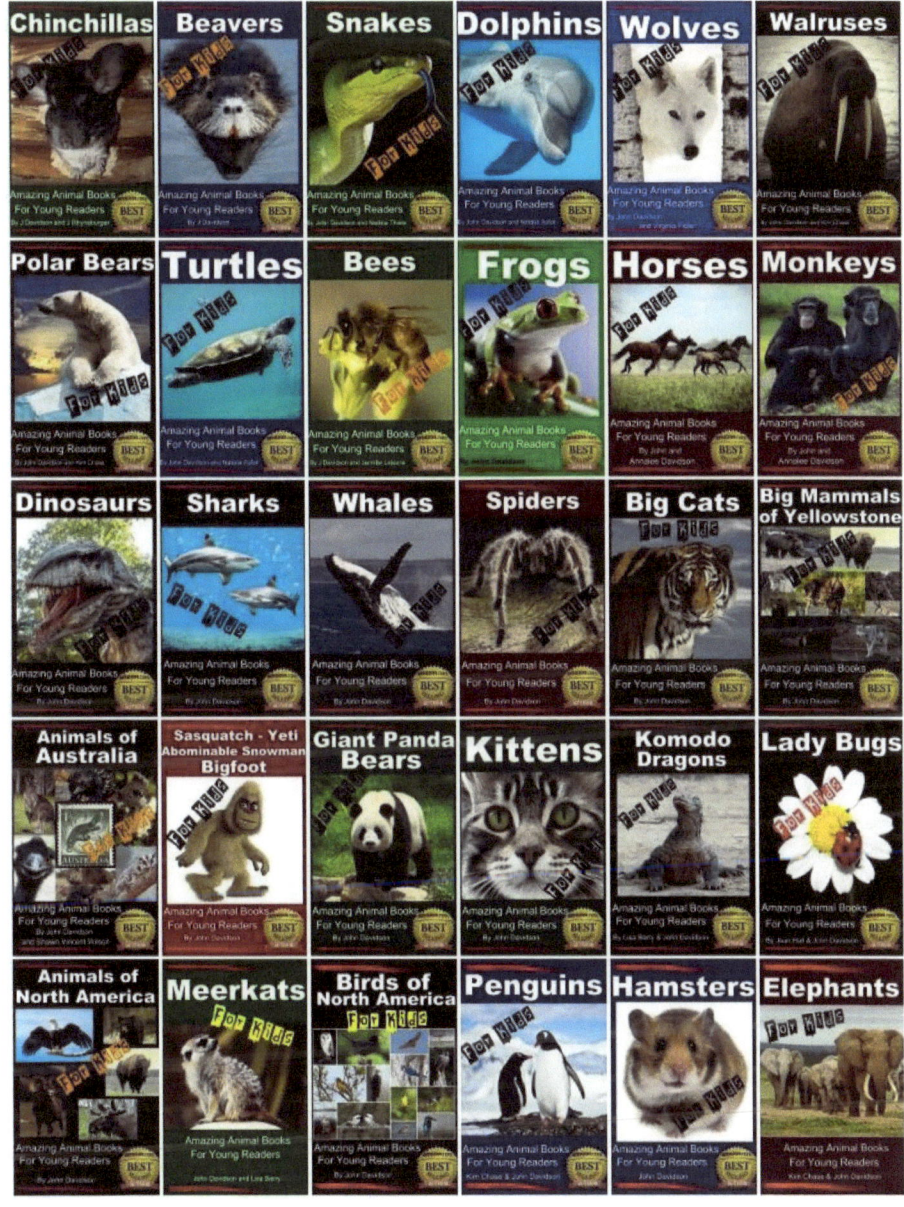

Learn To Draw Series

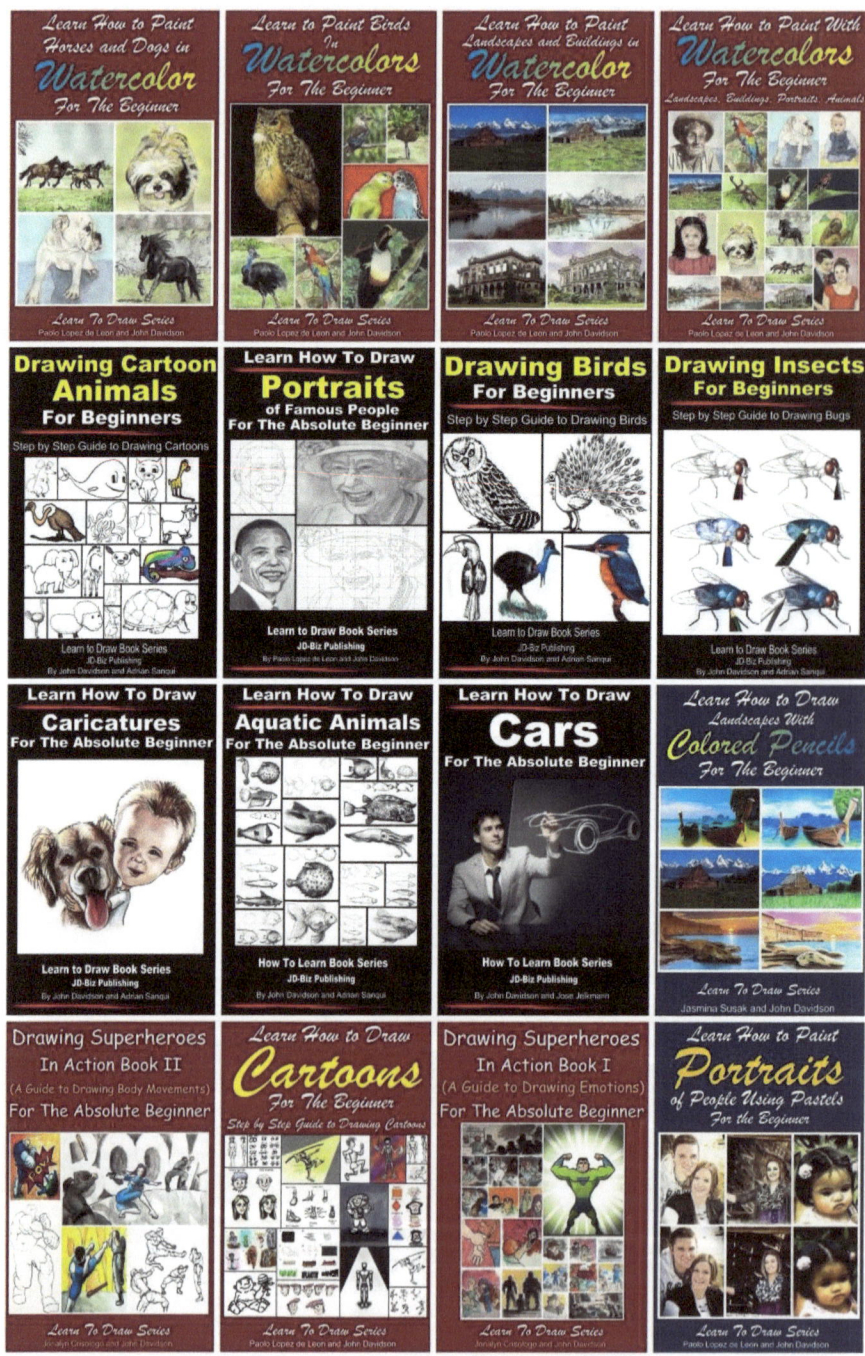

How to Build and Plan Books

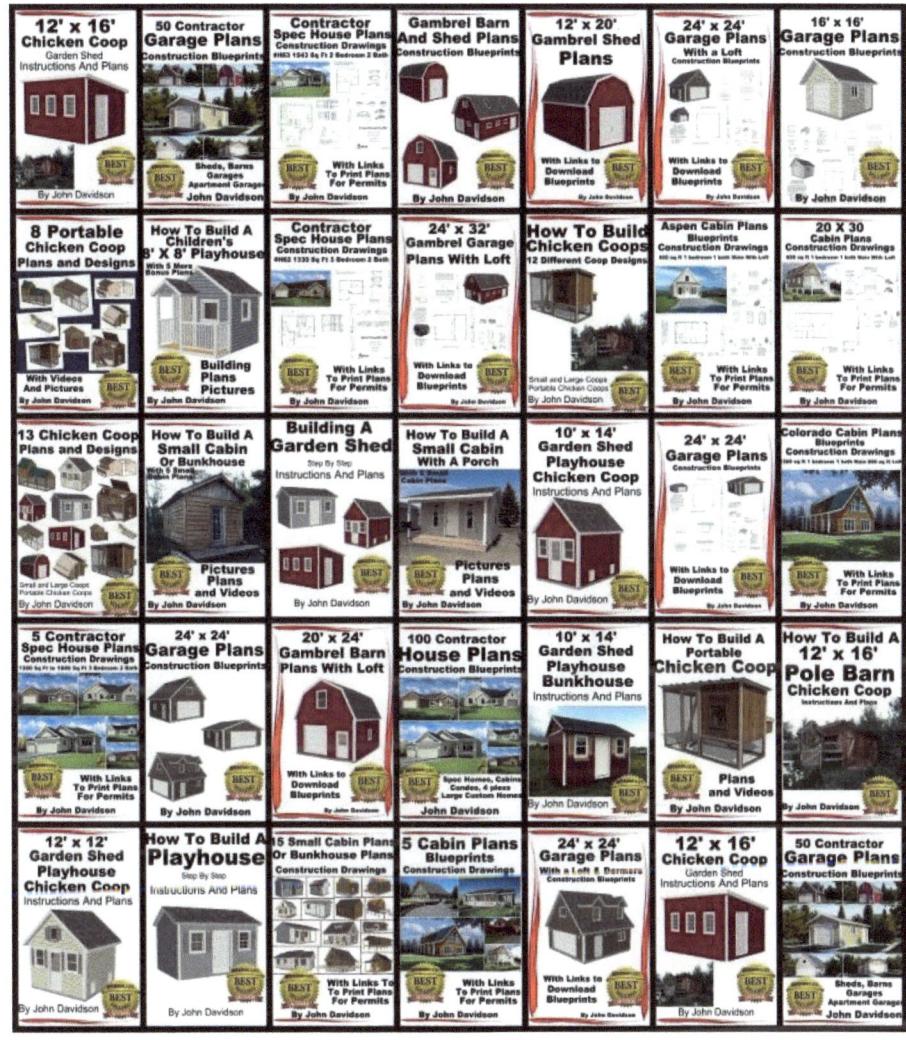

Entrepreneur Book Series

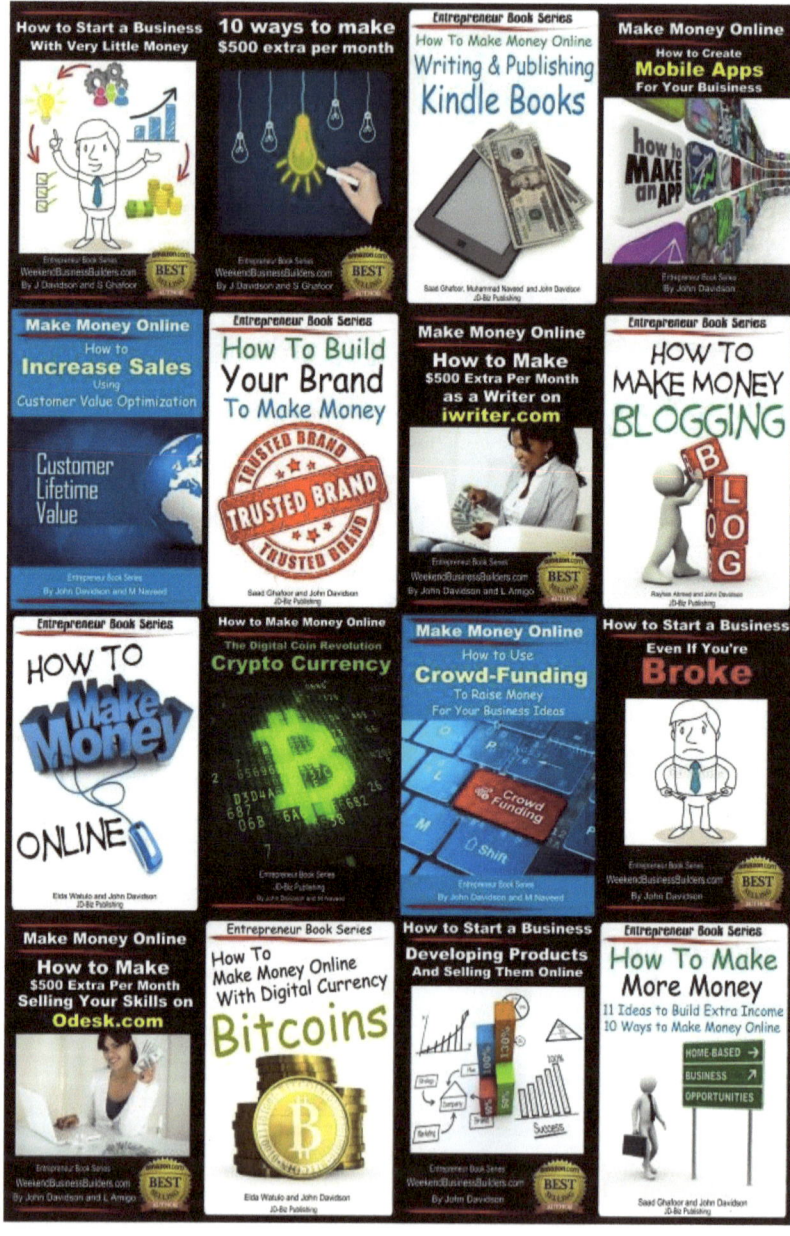

Our books are available at

1. Amazon.com
2. Barnes and Noble
3. Itunes
4. Kobo
5. Smashwords
6. Google Play Books

Download Free Books!
http://MendonCottageBooks.com

Publisher

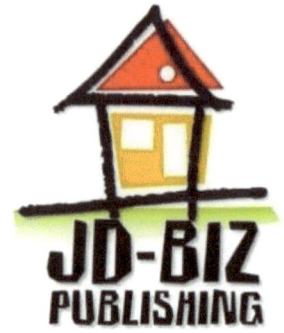

JD-Biz Corp

P O Box 374

Mendon, Utah 84325

http://www.jd-biz.com/

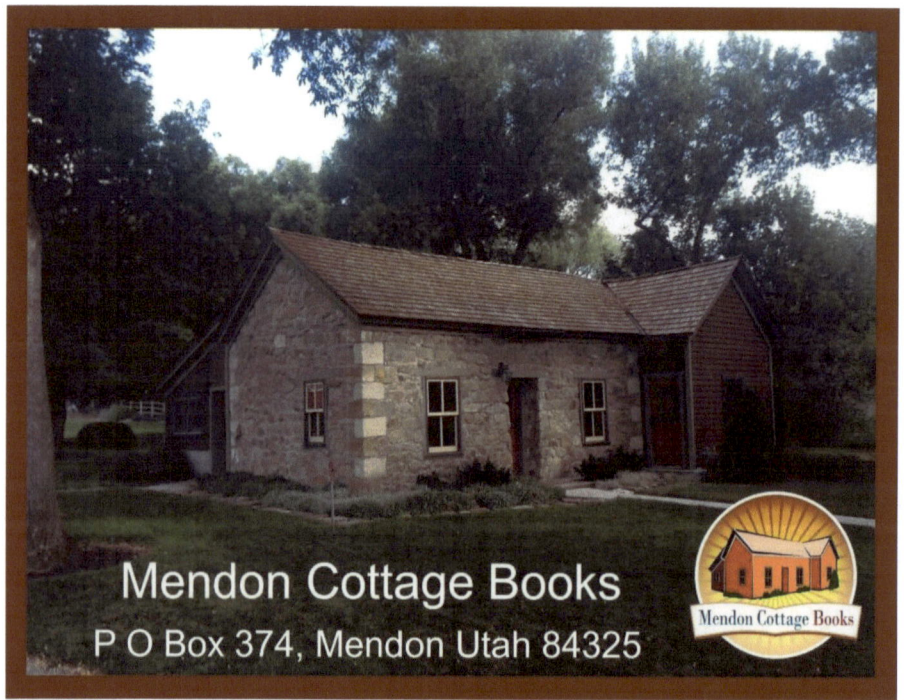

Mendon Cottage Books

P O Box 374, Mendon Utah 84325

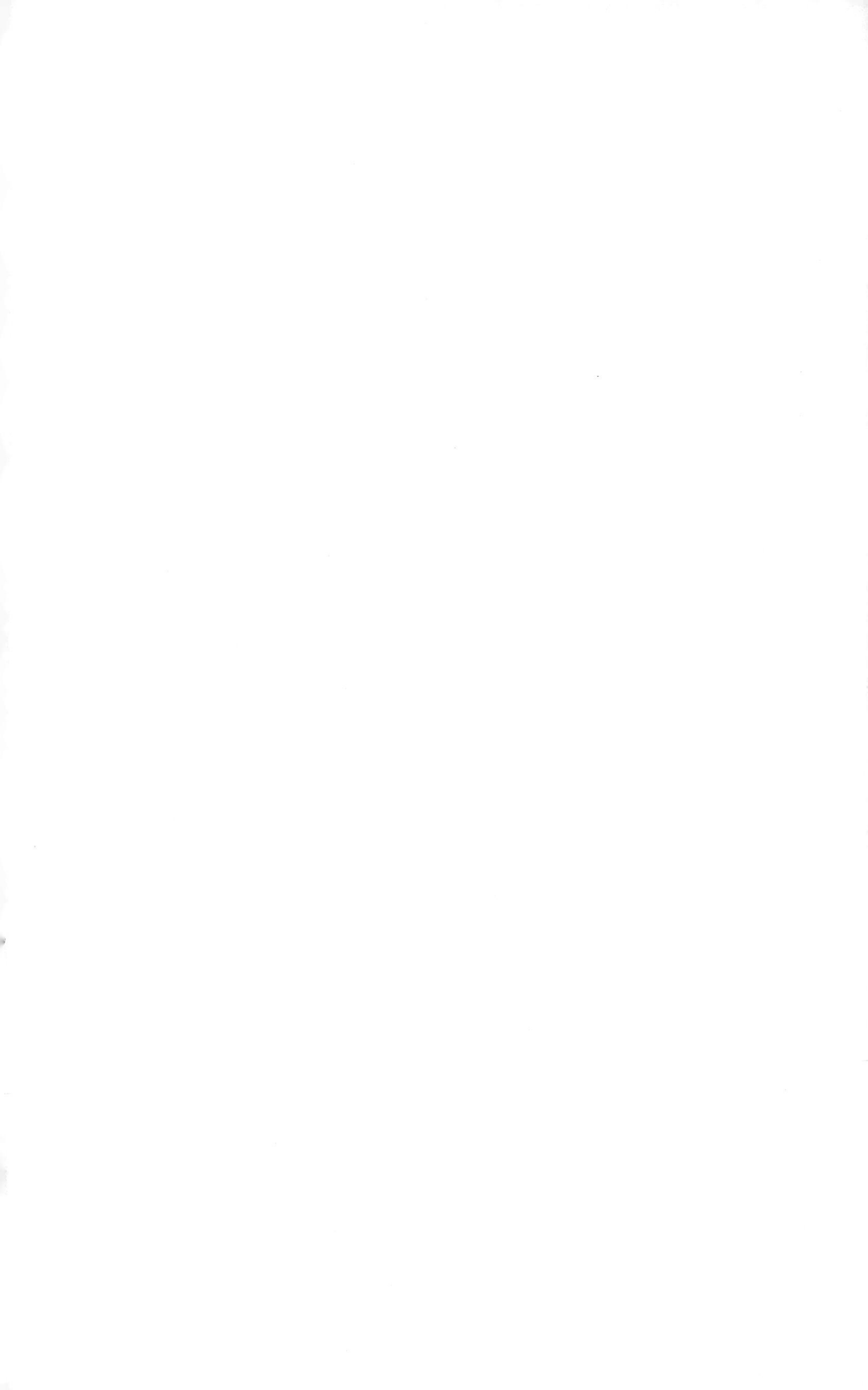

www.ingramcontent.com/pod-product-compliance
Lightning Source LLC
Chambersburg PA
CBHW040859180526
45159CB00001B/470